Laurene L Wright

Table of content

Conclusion

INTRODUCTION

Few experiences compare to the profoundly altering journey of motherhood in the broad scheme of existence. Every mother is an artist who uses unwavering love, resiliency, and unending devotion as her palette. She sets out on a journey that not only moulds her own personality but also the lives she affects. In "The Tunnel of light " the author explores the subtle nuances of this incredible journey, highlighting the highs and lows, challenges and joys, and complex strokes that come together to form the magnificent Canvas that is motherhood.

We will explore the nuances of pregnancy, delivery, and the delicate dance of balancing duties as we go through these pages. We'll take a peek inside the emotional rollercoaster that goes along with every kind grin, every achievement, and the silent times of introspection. This book tries to express the essence of the mother experience, from the fragility of infant beginnings to the tenacity needed in the face of parental hardships.

These chapters will examine how mother-child relationships have changed throughout time, creating a dynamic tapestry that is weaved together. Together, we'll overcome the difficulties of parenting teens, figure out how to handle the ups and downs of motherhood, and recognise and appreciate all of our accomplishments, no matter how minor. We will explore the successes of women who have confronted adversity with grace and come out of it as resilient artists who have created their own original Canvas through the prism of common experiences.

"The Tunnel of light" is more than simply a book; it's a celebration of the creativity that all mothers possess, an ode to the power that can be discovered in vulnerability, and an admission of the enormous influence moms have on the course of history. Together, let's explore the theme of motherhood via literature, where love has no boundaries and every chapter contributes to the construction of a timeless Canvas.

CHAPTER ONE

Pregnancy and expectations

Starting the amazing adventure of pregnancy is a life-changing event that takes place over the course of nine months of wonder. Every day brings a new life blossoming and the body going through significant changes, creating a tapestry of emotions, difficulties, and moments of pure amazement. Let's explore the many phases of this nine-month pregnant journey while honouring the wonders of infancy

- Months 1–3: Revealed Secret The first trimester is a subdued dance between eagerness and concealment. When a woman's body begins to grow the tiny seed of life, pregnancy begins to show symptoms. A deep change takes place within, even though it's veiled from the outside. An increase in hormones causes changes in the body as well as the emotions. Weakness, exhaustion, and sharpened senses accompany you on this enigmatic voyage.

- Months 4–6: The Bump That Blossoms As the second trimester approaches, the secret is happily revealed, and the world sees the first telltale symptoms of a growing baby: a blooming bump. The infant's feeling of connection develops along with it. The first flutters and kicks are exciting for parents, who treasure every ultrasound as a priceless window into the wonders of life. The onset of the mid-pregnancy glow eases the early discomforts.

- Months 7–9: The Last Mile There is a mixture of

excitement and expectation throughout the final trimester of pregnancy. The amazing trip is now evident in the tummy, and the baby's birth is quickly approaching. Parenting instincts take over as they get ready for the next phase of life. Physical discomforts resurface in the midst of the ecstasy, reminding the mother of the extraordinary fortitude required to bring a new life into the world.

NURTURING CHANGE

Embracing Transformation

Pregnancy is a period of emotional and psychological metamorphosis in addition to the physical changes. Emotions are strong, hormones change, and fresh viewpoints on life and family arise.

NURTURING BOND

Partners are essential in offering understanding and support throughout this emotional rollercoaster. Keeping the connection strong Throughout the nine months, the focus is not only on getting ready for the baby's birth but also on strengthening the link between the parents and the developing child within. Prenatal meal plans, book reading, and talking about goals and worries may all help to build a stronger bond between partners and a strong foundation for the adventure of parenthood to come. It is critical to look after one's physical and emotional well-being when pregnant. A balanced diet, frequent checkups, and physical activity are all beneficial to a healthy pregnancy. Furthermore, keeping lines of communication open with medical professionals guarantees that any issues are resolved quickly, creating a secure atmosphere for the mother and the child.

THE LAST COUNTDOWN

The Last Countdown Anxiety and a hint of excitement are in the air as the deadline draws near. The hospital bag that has been meticulously packed, the cot that is ready for its small baby, and the support system that is in place all contribute to the historic day that labour starts. The last push signifies the end of an amazing nine months of travel and the start of a new chapter in life, both physically and figuratively. Nine months of travel is a symphony of development, change, and expectation. Every instant provides evidence of the human body's tenacity and beauty, from its hidden origins to its outward manifestations. The nine-month pregnant journey is a monument to the wonder of life and the eternal fortitude of the human spirit, as parents excitedly await the arrival of their little one.

The Symphony of Birth

The nine-month pregnant journey stands as a tribute to the wonder of life and the enduring resilience of the human spirit.

The Birth Symphony. There was an air of expectation in the delivery room, with its clean white walls and the gentle buzz of medical equipment. Sarah lay in the middle of the stage, encased in a tornado of feelings. The adventure of pregnancy was coming to a culmination—a woven fabric of wonder and expectation.Each wave of the contractions appeared to convey the sounds of countless generations of women who had walked this hallowed route before them. Sarah's respiration synchronised with the monitor, creating a heartbeat that echoed both within and outside and linked her to the pulsating pulse of existence.Dr. Reynolds was a comforting presence to Sarah during her labour, a light of calm in the midst of the storm. A quiet orchestra of skilled hands and sympathetic eyes made up the medical staff surrounding her. Every participant in the birth symphony performed a specific instrument, such as the midwife's gentle whispers, the obstetrician's measured instructions, or the nurses' swaying dance.Sarah had a significant metamorphosis as she gave in to the agony and resolved. The room was transformed from a clinical setting to a vehicle for life's spectacular blossoming. With every contraction, she got closer to the moment that would mark the conclusion of months of waiting—

the time when mother and child's worlds would finally connect.Sarah took comfort in the group of people around her throughout the worst part of labour. The nurses were like guardian angels, helping her through the storm with their kind words and touches. The birthing process was like a complex dance, requiring not just physical stamina but also an unwavering spirit.A final burst of vitality caused the room to explode with sounds, including a newborn's scream, the relief breaths of doctors, and Sarah's victorious sigh. As Dr. Reynolds gently held the little creature, time appeared to stop still. This work of art was created from the very essence of life.During the brief moment before the infant found comfort in Sarah's arms, the room was eerily silent. A holy interval before the world acknowledged the entrance of a new soul, the stillness carried the weight of the supernatural. The sound of the baby's screams had previously been a tune of doubt, but now it held the promise of an unknown future.A wave of feelings swept through Sarah as the baby pressed itself to her chest: a wave of love, wonder, and an overpowering sense of duty. Mother and kid had a quiet discussion in those first few seconds of the meeting. Their gaze met, and in one glance, a bond was established that was weaved throughout their common life.The space had been electrified with the intensity of work, but it was now a peaceful haven. This private dance between mother and child was allowed to continue since the medical staff stood aside. Once the room's steady pulse was established, the monitors now provided a calm background for the conversations—

a comforting lullaby amid the quiet.The profoundness of birth persisted in the days that followed as the family adapted to the ups and downs of a newborn's requirements. With every day that went by, the baby—a small traveller in a big universe—started to show its true nature. Together with James, her boyfriend, Sarah negotiated the unfamiliar seas of motherhood, finding comfort in the trials and moments of delight they had together.The story of their family was shaped by the tremendous experience of giving birth and the first few minutes of getting to know the infant. A life created from the depths of Sarah's existence, a witness to the remarkable ability of the human body and spirit, amazed her as she held the baby in her arms in the silence of the night.Sarah took on the role of storyteller as the delivery chapter developed, incorporating her experiences into the tapestry of family history. The delivery room, which had previously served as a platform for the birth's symphony, was now a treasured memory and a hallowed area where the common and exceptional came together to dance through eternity.Up until now, the voyage had been a tapestry of feelings, including excitement, anticipation, and maybe a hint of fear. Throughout her pregnancy, Sarah experienced both emotional and physical development. The bond between mother and child had grown stronger, beginning with the first fluttering kicks that indicated life within and continuing through the quiet times she would spend cradling her growing belly.

CHAPTER TWO

Early Days of Motherhood

The First Motherhood Years It is nearly impossible to describe becoming a mother. You know what to expect, including plenty of cuddles from the baby, less sleep, and pain while you heal from giving birth. But you'll be surprised by a few things as well! These are some of the things you should anticipate or probably encounter.

1. You join a new tribe right away. You automatically join a network of women who have been in similar situations before the moment your child is born. And nothing compares to the support that other mothers can provide! All of them have experienced similar things, and the majority of them are just eager to share their wisdom with incoming

"mom tribe" members. Lean on them for support, ask them questions about what worked best for them, and know that you're not alone on this new adventure into motherhood. One excellent strategy to manage and process the early transition to parenthood is to join a postpartum group. It may also be a source of comfort and reassurance to connect with other moms and realise that you are not alone in your struggles and experiences as a new mother, even if you might be reluctant to meet new people while you already have so much on your plate.

2. It Could Be Difficult to "Switch Off" Being the one in charge of this adorable, delicate little child might be thrilling, but it can also cause some anxiety. For several weeks after bringing their newborns home, several mothers are taken aback by

how different they feel from their "normal" selves. Perhaps it's the protective mother bear in new mothers, but anxiety over whether you're doing the right thing and that your child is safe and well can set you on edge. When the infant is asleep, this uneasy feeling can be more upsetting. Although it's common knowledge to "sleep when a baby sleeps," some new mothers find it difficult to unwind and feel awake all the time, even when they're tired. When their infant is sound asleep, some new parents have even reported hearing "phantom cries." Usually, these nervous sensations subside in a few weeks as you become more accustomed to your new position. It's crucial to get in touch with your healthcare practitioner if you have excessive worries or anxieties, hopelessness, sorrow, guilt, anger, anxiety, or a sense of losing control for more than two weeks. While mood swings are common among new moms, 15-20% of them also report more severe symptoms of anxiety or postpartum depression.

3. You Might Not Want Guests You might have imagined inviting loved ones to your house to meet your new baby before you had the baby. It may surprise you to learn that you don't want anyone to visit in the weeks after the baby is born, save for your or your partner's parents. Remember, when the time is appropriate for you, you can introduce your baby to your friends and family in the upcoming weeks and months. Before accepting offers for guests, talk with your spouse or support person about your needs and expectations. Assign yourself or your support team to act as the gatekeeper, declining visits and

telling people to leave when you're ready for them to stop. By doing this, you may spare yourself the trouble of breaking the news and let someone else bear the mental and emotional burden of early fatherhood. The early days of a newborn's life fly by. It might feel rather daunting to have a house full of people to entertain on top of recuperating from birth, understanding your baby's feeding signals, and trying to get some sleep. And it's alright! Tell anyone who requests a visit that you're just not ready for them at this time, and you'll let them know when they can come by. Establishing appropriate boundaries gives you the time and space you need to recover and form bonds with your infant, even if you may be afraid of failing your friends and family.

4.It's Not Always Intuitive to Breastfeed While many new mothers initially intend to breastfeed, some are taken aback to learn that it's not always easy. While some infants and their mothers may easily get into the swing of nursing, for others it may require some time, patience, and a genuine test of a new mother's will. Acknowledging that breastfeeding can be more difficult than popular belief might help eliminate any sense of surprise and instill the belief that mastering a new skill requires patience. For your child and yourself.

5. You may sweat and experience body odour. After giving birth, your body could do some unexpected things, including start perspiring more than normal and develop body odour. Hormone changes can throw your body into a loop, much like when you go through puberty.

While some body odour can be attributed to changes in hormone levels, breastfeeding is also a contributing factor in these strange scents. The vision of a newborn is not very excellent. As a result, new moms really release several pheromones that might assist in cueing your baby to suckle at the breast. Sweating is how it works to get rid of these additional fluids. Sweat is especially noticeable to some mothers at night. Investing in a waterproof mattress pad is a smart move to prevent your mattress from being ruined by nighttime perspiration.

6. It may take some time to fall in love with your baby. Every mother who has ever given birth probably experiences the first time she sees her child in a different way. Some people could experience wonder. Astonishment might be felt by

some. Like in the movies, some people may fall madly in love the instant their child is born. However, surprise! You're not alone if you're not a mother who feels this overwhelming, unconditional love right away. Some mothers require time to heal, adjust, and get to know their newborn due to the process of giving birth and the sudden change in identity. Never undervalue the importance of treating oneself with kindness and gentleness. Talk to your spouse, friends, and family about how they can help you throughout the early stages of motherhood, if at all feasible. Mama, don't worry if you don't fall completely in love with your child right away. It's going to happen. Although every mother experiences things at a different time, it's normal for these things to take time. You'll get there if you spend skin-to-skin time, make eye contact, and give your infant cuddles.

7. You Could Lose Your Pre-Baby Years If you've always wanted a child of your own, you might be surprised to discover that after you're a parent, you miss some aspects of your "old life." It's also critical to understand that this does not imply ungraciousness. A significant change in identity, routines, energy levels, and the flexibility to do as you want, whenever you like, comes with being a mother. It's acceptable to acknowledge that life has changed and become more difficult. Recognise the reality of the changes in your life, concentrate on the positive aspects of this new you, and realise that you are most certainly not the only one who feels this way. Additionally, keep in mind that as your child gets older, the demands

on your time and attention will also vary. Even if your pre-baby lifestyle does not return, you will have more time and energy to take up some of your favourite pastimes and activities.

8. You and your companion must regain your footing. It will take some getting used to your new duties as parents for you and your spouse. Furthermore, although it would be ideal if both spouses could seamlessly transition into their new roles and responsibilities, this is frequently not the case. It may be stressful and intimidating to become a new parent. When you combine it with insufficient sleep, even the most stable of couples could find themselves having more arguments and annoyance than they bargained for. greatest advice, Try to communicate with each other in an honest and straightforward manner.

Instead of allowing your wants, disappointments, and emotions to fester, talk to each other about them. This makes sure that in the early stages of parenting, you

ADAPTING TO MOTHERHOOD'S DIFFICULTIES

initial Pregnancy and motherhood are transformative times. In reaction to these changes, new parents frequently feel a range of emotions, both happy and sad. Pregnancy and childbirth are often more difficult than individuals had imagined; this is a typical readjusting experience. But for some, the difficulties become too much to bear. It's critical to get assistance when this happens. Numerous community and health resources are available to help, and there are numerous personal stress-reduction strategies you may try.

DIFFICULTIES NEW PARENTS FACE

- fatigue from adjusting to a rigorous sleep and feeding schedule
- The physical demands of nursing include mastitis, broken nipples, and discomfort when latching on.
- recuperation after delivery while taking care of a newborn
- The challenges of meeting your wants and those of your infant while managing a home.
- Lack of faith in your capacity to comprehend the demands of the infant.
- Managing the demands and guidance from loved ones and friends.
- Personal identity transformation: this might

involve losing your job and its associated prestige, your social life, and your sense of independence.

- Relationship modifications with your spouse might involve addressing different parenting philosophies, as well as adjustments to your needs and attitude towards physical closeness.

- An additional baby means a change in the dynamics of the family.

A sentimental moment

It can be emotionally taxing to care for a newborn during the first few weeks and months. The emotional ups and downs might be perplexing; it takes some getting used to being a mother. Your emotional state may be influenced by pain, fatigue, your birth story, and the level of assistance you get. The sensation of being on an emotional roller coaster may intensify if your expectations and the reality of being a mother diverge. In addition to the "baby blues," most women often have days when they feel overburdened by the task of taking care of a newborn.

The advice and methods for navigating through

- Learn about and cherish your child. Initially, the task of taking care of a newborn around-the-clock might be rather demanding.
- Try to unwind; you'll quickly find out what he likes and needs. Accepting and providing for a newborn's demand for intimacy is the simplest approach to take care of him. You'll see subtle patterns starting to emerge after some time. From there, you may expand on these

patterns to establish a daily routine that works for you both.

- To obtain better sleep, bring your infant into your room or onto your bed. And what about older kids and domestic duties?

Some women prepare ahead of time and request help with daily housework, child care, and food and snack preparation.

- Accepting assistance from friends helps reduce stress.

Accepting offers of assistance may be made simpler if a list of easy activities is prepared.

- For important jobs, reserve your energy. Not every household task is equally significant.

CHAPTER THREE

INFANT BLUE

A minor, transient ailment known as "baby blues" is linked to the hormone levels in the body dropping after delivery. After giving birth, between 30 and 85 percent of new moms report having "baby blues," which typically begin three to five days later. Some women endure mood swings, bewilderment, forgetfulness, migraines, unfavourable attitudes towards the infant, restlessness, impatience, and nightmares. Some mothers just discover that they cry spontaneously. Thankfully, this illness usually passes within a few days.Early on

- Rest and sleep: You have just completed a tremendous task by developing and giving birth to your child, so it's critical that you allow yourself permission to rest and sleep. Aim for a minimum of one or two weeks to allow for recuperation.

- Breastfeed frequently: Having a newborn and breastfeeding together releases calming chemicals that are meant to ease your anxiety in the early going. On the other hand, strict scheduling may increase stress.

- Hug your child: Try Biological NurturingTM; "laid back" postures can help you feel calmer and more secure during nursing.

- Spend time together: You might want to set up a cosy space with enough privacy so that you and your child can spend a lot of time together.

- Visitor cap: Limiting guests is OK; you may write "new mum and baby resting, please call back in a few days" on your door or urge your husband to explain that you're exhausted. Visitors are less inclined to remain longer and could even bring you a cup of tea if you are in your dressing gown or are in bed with your infant.
- Prepare in advance: To ensure that you are able to sleep without being interrupted, use an answerphone or put your phone on quiet.

DEPRESSION

It's critical that you speak with your doctor or health visitor if any of the unfavourable emotions worsen or persist longer than two weeks, such as if you experience overwhelm, worry, or difficulty falling asleep. It is not unusual for new moms to experience depression, and there is a wealth of resources available to support these mothers and their children. Moms can recuperate rapidly with the right care and can then completely enjoy becoming parents to their newborn.

There are medications on the market that are safe to take while nursing. You may get information Professionals on which medications are safe to use while nursing, get in touch with a local LLL breastfeeding counsellor, or get assistance by calling our National Telephone Helpline. Homestart is a nationwide nonprofit organisation that provides companionship and support to families with young children who are experiencing difficulties managing for any kind of cause.

Get moving around:

Sunshine and fresh air are beneficial to your health. Most moms realise how important it is to work out every day to improve their happiness; in the early weeks, even a quick five- to ten-minute stroll can help. Going out with your child can also provide structure for your day and keep you from feeling alone. Soon, you'll be able to take your infant on trips to the neighbourhood park, library, and stores. However, don't try too hard or too quickly. Work up slowly. You might also begin engaging in enjoyable, mild activities like singing, swimming, or baby massage with other women and their infants.

Take care of yourself:

Consuming sensible foods, such as wholesome snacks, can have an impact. Consuming a diet rich in wholegrain bread and cereals, pasta, potatoes, rice, vegetables, legumes, and fresh fruits may help maintain stable blood sugar levels, warding off exhaustion and sadness. Eating a diet rich in long-chain omega-3 fatty acids, EPA and DHA, can help you manage stress and perhaps stave off depression. Rich meals and oily seafood are examples of sources. Should you be thinking about using supplements, speak with your physician. Stay hydrated by drinking enough water to maintain a light urine colour. Both water and a daily glass of fruit juice are beneficial. Refrain from consuming alcohol, caffeine, and carbonated beverages. You can have better sleep if you eat meals high in complex carbs, milk, or bananas before bed. When your kid is sleeping, give yourself the attention you need and attend to your own needs, such as rest and sleep. When you have a few minutes, employ the relaxation methods you may have learned for labour. You should schedule some alone time for yourself. Take a bath or shower, read a magazine or book, or watch a DVD while nursing your child. Postnatal activities are excellent, but avoid over-exerting oneself. Negative emotions might be exacerbated by pain and fatigue.

Engage in social interactions:

It can help to spend time with other mothers, whether in person or virtually.

Both our online Facebook groups and local LLL meetings are excellent places to meet other nursing mothers. All parents may also get information and help from Children and Family Centres located all around the nation.

Any breastfeeding issues should be addressed right once since suffering in silence may depress you greatly.

Why not have a conversation with a sympathetic person? Talking about your feelings might help you come up with coping mechanisms.

Since it's not always simple for others to understand what you're going through, try to communicate your needs to your spouse. Hugs, handshakes, and encouraging remarks may make a big difference.

Try to pay attention to your body as time passes and adjust your exercise level to match your current state of energy. There will always be days when your child gets older when it's a good idea to take a nap or sleep while your child is sleeping. It takes a lot of effort to keep up with a crawling newborn or an energetic toddler.

Remind yourself that your baby needs and loves you when you're feeling down. Embrace him tightly. He only needs you; he doesn't need a flawless mother. Additionally, you are significant.

Give yourself time so that experience can teach you. Avoid severely judging yourself based on what other people expect of you.

Developing a relationship with the infant

- Bonding and attachment are about responding to your newborn baby's needs with love, warmth, and care. You become your baby's special, trusted person when you act in this way on a regular basis. Why developing a bond with infants is vital The formation of a bond between you and your newborn is essential to their growth. Your baby feels the world is a safe place to play, learn, and explore when they get from you the things they need, such as a smile, a touch, or a cuddle. This lays the groundwork for growth and well-being during infancy. Moreover, bonding promotes your baby's

- physical and mental development. For instance, your baby's brain releases hormones when you touch, cuddle, converse, sing, and look each other in the eyes on a regular basis. These hormones enable your baby's brain to expand. Additionally, as their brain develops, your child begins to acquire language, cognition, and memory. Not only does plenty of snuggle time and skin-to-skin contact promote bonding,

- Additionally, it calms infants down, lessens crying, and improves their sleep. Recognising the bonding behaviours of newborns When your infant wants to bond with you and deepen your relationship, they let you know through body language. For instance, your child may grunt or look you in the eye. Make little sounds, like coos or laughter, to convey your attention and relaxation. Your kid feels confident when you pay attention to their indications and body language and respond in a warm and caring manner. Additionally
- , it encourages your kid to communicate more and helps

them learn about social behaviour, emotions, and communication. It's all part of strengthening your bond.

The Art of Juggling:

Handling the Various Demands of Motherhood With all of its benefits and drawbacks, motherhood is a complex path. A woman enters a stage when balancing obligations becomes a daily performance the minute she accepts the job of mother. The complexities of perfecting this art are examined in this chapter, which also examines the abilities, difficulties, and coping mechanisms that characterise the juggling act of motherhood

I. The Various Functions of Motherhood Being a mother requires taking on several duties. Mothers have many different and difficult obligations, ranging from taking care of a baby to handling domestic matters. She starts the balancing act by switching between being her child's carer, teacher, and emotional support system with ease.

II. The Infant Stage: An Upheaval of Accountability Early on in parenting, the juggling act becomes more difficult. It becomes normal to have restless nights, to feed continuously, and to comfort a screaming baby. Even the most seasoned mothers find it difficult to juggle their own demands and domestic obligations with a newborn's urgent requirements.

III. Juggling Motherhood and Work The balancing act for a lot of moms goes outside the house. A careful balance must be struck while juggling the demands of parenthood and employment obligations. Having supportive work environments, flexible work schedules, and maternity leave are crucial for preserving a healthy balance between work and family life.

IV. Caring for Hearts and Minds via Emotional Labour Motherhood is more than just physical labour; emotional labour is an important part of it. Providing a safe emotional foundation, teaching values, and guiding a kid through emotional landscapes are all essential to a child's growth yet frequently go unacknowledged. V. Collaborating in Parenting When you share the juggling act with someone else, it becomes more sustainable. Co-parenting entails working together to share duties, make decisions, and offer emotional support. Couples that support and understand one another better are able to work through the challenges of parenting a child as a team. VI. Obstacles and

Giving Up Motherhood is an art of juggling, not without its difficulties and sacrifices. Mothers often have to choose between their own goals and their children's needs. The pressure from society to live up to inflated expectations makes the juggling act much more difficult.

VII. Techniques for Effective Juggling Motherhood is a balancing act that takes a toolkit of methods to navigate successfully. Task prioritisation, efficient communication, and time management become essential skills. Mothers may preserve balance without sacrificing their wellbeing by learning how to delegate tasks both at home and at work.

VIII. Taking Care of Oneself Is an Absolute Priority In the middle of all the obligations, self-care becomes an absolute must. Mothers need to understand how critical it is to support their mental and physical health. Maintaining resilience in the juggling act requires setting aside time for introspection, rest, and pursuit of personal interests. Look for allies and role models. There is no requirement for a formal reporting arrangement. Look for role models who embody the qualities you want in your life. I am honoured to know and call my working mom advisors at West Monroe, where there are so many powerful women in leadership roles. Men have also put in a lot of effort to help me get the jobs and projects I want in the company. Inquire about their experience and the steps they take to keep themselves happy both at work and at home. You'll be astonished by how willing people are to assist you and how honest they will be once you start a conversation.

IX. Establishing a Safety Net When moms create a strong network of support, the idea of the village becomes more apparent. The support systems of friends, family, and the community provide moms with the ability to manage their tasks more skillfully. The strains of juggling are lessened by shared obligations and experiences. It's part of the job to compromise. It is unlikely that you will be able to attend every evening networking event and every happy hour. Use your time wisely, and choose your activities carefully. You are not required to do something just because you want to. You will eventually be free from concern over this trade-off, but for now, accept it and go on.

X. Rejoicing in the Face of Responsibilities It is important for moms to take a moment to appreciate the blessings of parenting in the middle of the juggling act. These moments, which range from a child's first grin to their accomplishments, serve as reminders of the beauty that comes along with the difficulties of juggling. The skill of balancing obligations while becoming a mother is a dynamic, continuing process. Mothers create a masterpiece characterised by love, resiliency, and unshakable dedication as they skillfully negotiate the complex dance of life's demands. The juggling act, with all of its benefits and challenges, adds to the beautiful tapestry of motherhood, demonstrating the grace and strength that each mother possesses.

CHAPTER FOUR

Mental Health Services

It may be particularly difficult for new mothers to recognise when they are suffering due to the widespread stigma in our society around mental health. New mothers face societal expectations that are too high. When a baby is born, moms should be overjoyed. Feelings of panic, anxiety, despair, or being overwhelmed should have no place in your life. On the other hand, this is completely unnecessary and wrong. Mothers are the backbone of our society, and we can all do more to help them. To begin, let's clarify a few words. It is normal for a woman to go through a wide range of emotions after giving birth since her body goes through so many changes. Within the first few weeks after giving birth, new mothers may go through a period of emotional instability, weeping spells, anxiety, and trouble sleeping, which is referred to as the "baby blues." Nonetheless, some parents may feel more severe, long-lasting sorts of concern or sadness termed postpartum depression (PPD) or anxiety (PPA). PPA and PPD don't hint to defects in character or weakness. They are a message from your body that it needs greater assistance during the postpartum period. Symptoms and indications The symptoms of postpartum depression may vary. While baby blues and PPD symptoms could be confused for one another at first, PPD symptoms are generally more severe and long-lasting. The uncomfortable sensations Being a mother is a fantastic experience that comes with a lot of responsibility, deep love, and emotional ups and downs for women. A complex and dynamic emotional landscape is generated when the lows of worries and self-doubt are coupled with the highs of extraordinary happenings. This chapter covers the complexities of the dramatic emotional rollercoaster that is becoming a mother, offering insight on the enormous spectrum of sensations that accompany this transforming event.

I. Excitement and Expectation The first step on the emotional rollercoaster that is parenting is the excitement of a new life. An ultrasound picture, a positive pregnancy test, and the first fluttering kicks may produce conflicting feelings, ranging from intense delight to a hint of dread. Emotions are a big component of the experience as soon as the trip starts.

II. The Incredible Arrival: Joy and Chaos As labour continues on, the emotional rollercoaster reaches its pinnacle. When a mother sees her kid for the first time, she may experience a multitude of feelings, such as wonder, unconditional love, and possibly an overpowering sense of duty. Early motherhood is marked by a unique blend of feelings that are produced from a combination of happiness and tiredness.

III. The Sleepless Nights: Comfort and Fatigue The hardships of taking care of a baby give birth to a whole new gamut of emotions. Sleepless nights, continuous feedings, and continually caring to a screaming newborn test a mother's stamina. As tiredness sets in, there are moments of immense affection for the infant intermingled with periods of pure exhaustion.

IV. Finding a Balance: Handling Accountabilities and Opinions Moms undergo a more intense emotional rollercoaster as they manage their obligations. Balancing the requirements of the child, taking care of domestic tasks, and, for some, pursuing a profession all contribute to the construction of a tapestry of emotions. These feelings run from times of uncertainty and sorrow to pleasure with one's achievements.

V. The Joys of Milestones: Pride and Memories Every developmental milestone is coupled with a new emotional high. When their children walk, smile, or speak for the first time, moms are overwhelmed with enormous pride. There's also a sense of sorrow and a feeling that time is going by too rapidly. Section VI:

VI. The Emotional Labour: Taking Good Care of Hearts and Minds The emotional rollercoaster that is motherhood's emotional travail occurs beyond the concrete facts. As they follow their children through emotional ups and downs, teach values, and offer consolation, moms go through a significant emotional journey. 7. Difficulties and

VII. Self-Doubt: The Rollercoaster's Deep End When presented with problems, whether in the shape of behavioural disorders, health concerns, or social limitations, mothers go through the lowest periods of the emotional rollercoaster. Feelings of despair, discontent, and a strong want for affirmation occur as self-doubt takes hold.

VIII. The Strength of the Assistance: Rebounding Support systems help the emotional rollercoaster stay balanced when faced with obstacles. Moms need the help of friends, family, and partners to regain mental stability and get through difficult times.

IX. Striking a Balance: Using Self-Care to Restore Stem Cells Mothers who realise the benefits of emotional wellness start down the path to self-care. Taking up hobbies, setting aside time for introspection, and seeking periods of seclusion all become crucial resilience strategies while facing emotional ups and downs.

X. The Evolution of the Mother-Child Bond: An enchanting and intricate connection The emotional rollercoaster changes with time. The mother-child bond changes as time goes on, and the emotional terrain becomes more complex. The path from childhood to maturity is characterised by a blend of pride, anxiety, and deep, long-lasting love. Accepting the Exciting Adventure Maternity is an emotional rollercoaster, a complex journey with highs and lows that define the core of what it is to be a mother. Mothers who follow this route find an inner source of strength. Accepting the whole range of feelings, from exuberant highs to difficult lows, becomes a crucial component of the exquisite tapestry that is motherhood. Signs and feelings of depression Having given birth, experiencing helplessness severe mood swings and an overwhelming number of tears Sleep deprivation remorse, inadequacy, or humiliation It's difficult to form a relationship with your child, and you put friends and family at a distant. incapable of focusing, reasoning clearly, or drawing

Conclusion extreme anxiety, panic attacks, or a desire to hurt your child or yourself Postpartum depression is not something you have to deal with alone! The Emotional Volcano's Causes Following Childbirth But why was giving birth such a roller coaster of emotions? Hormones are the simple explanation. Hormone production in women's bodies increases throughout pregnancy and sharply declines after birth. Hormonal changes may contribute to moodiness, anxiety, melancholy, anger, and tension. In addition to regulating many other aspects of life, hormones also regulate metabolism, stress levels, sleep cycles, brain activity, and digestive health! It's not always that simple, however. The following other variables may potentially have an impact on the emotional rollercoaster that follows childbirth: genetics. Hormone fluctuations may be more prone to affect us due to our genetic makeup. previous mental health problems. Expectant moms with a history of depression are more likely to have PPD. recuperation Being a parent is the hardest thing you have ever done. It might be challenging, and recovery takes time! blood sugar instability Mothers often eat on the go, at odd hours, or not at all. Significant blood sugar fluctuations result from this, and they have an impact on mood, worry, weariness, and sadness. problems with sleeping. Is it difficult for you to get asleep, remain asleep, or wake up and go back to sleep after the baby? The state of our physical, mental, and emotional health is influenced by the calibre of our sleep. Guidance for Control After giving birth, these suggestions can make you feel more at ease emotionally.

Advice for mothers who don't have assistance

1. Establish a neighbourhood. Seeking assistance from others is OK! Friends, neighbours, coworkers, and family want to support you, but they're not sure how or where to start. Make every effort to request what you want when you require it. The amount of support your community has for you could surprise you.

2. Create a personal space. This is really crucial! Mothers, I strongly advise scheduling self-care activities and setting up a routine that will help you feel refreshed. I realise it's difficult and requires effort. Recall that the family's overall health

improves when mother gets the attention she need.

3. Moving Every day, move your body in ways that you like. A brief 20-minute stroll or dance party may lift your spirits, reduce tension, and return insulin and glucose levels to normal. Just be cautious not to push yourself too far.

4. Go to bed. This is easier said than done, I know! Everything in our life is better when we get more sleep. Take that snooze while the baby sleeps. Alternatively, offer to have a friend or neighbour keep the baby so that you may get some rest. Make it a goal to go to bed fifteen minutes earlier every night this week. Random information may be quite helpful.

5. Utilise screen time when you have breaks. In actuality, when you don't have a community or support system, you don't have much time to

yourself. In actuality, screen time is the simplest method to take a break when you have none else. It's been unfairly made into a villain. Screens are engaging, no question about it. There are a multitude of additional options accessible in addition to Netflix and Youtube, such as Reading Eggs and Khan Academy for Kids, among many more educational games. Furthermore, your child's excessive screen time need not be ongoing, despite your concerns. You can still include screen time into their daily routine even if you are an engaged parent who lets kids play outside. You're a capable mother. In fact, you'll most likely come back from your hiatus a stronger person.

6. Lower your expectations If you're looking for a parenting tip, this is the one that will change your game! It is suitable in any circumstance.

Meal times. How much work you wish to put in every day. The appearance of your kid as they walk out of the home. How often you clean up? The quality of your laundry folding. To what extent do you volunteer at the school where your kids attend? There is an infinite list. Simply said, you can't do everything, and trying to do so will just increase your stress levels. By following the adage "done is better than perfect" and marking things off your list, you will be able to prioritise yourself and create more opportunities for self-care.

7. Make plans to engage in playtime. If you plan out the times of day that you will be playing with your children, you can feel less guilty about the times that you are not. Although it is a myth that children should play actively with us all day, you may nevertheless

include them in cooking and other home tasks. Apart from self-care, you could also have a job to do and a house to maintain.

8. Save some cash for yourself. Out of all the advice for parents, this is my particular favourite. Stop squandering money on the kids, stop apologising, and quit feeling self-conscious about everything you buy for yourself, girl. Get yourself something instead. You deserve to have it. Your kids already have more than they need, for the most part. Maybe it's a new outfit, a fancy coffee while running errands, or sometimes getting your nails done. It's OK to indulge yourself without feeling bad about it. Because your kids are clinging to you, are you running short on time? Buy today and give yourself a pleasure.

9. Employers If you can afford it, hire someone to take care of the

chores you don't want to or don't have time to do in order to free up more time for the things you do want to get done. It may be anything: a dog walker, someone to shovel the driveway, a babysitter, a maid, a laundry service, someone to drop your child off to creche, etc. Investing a little sum of money to get more time might out to be quite advantageous. Getting your child to stay at creche for an extra hour can help you have more time for yourself after work. The secret is to figure out how to carve out time that doesn't appear to exist right now.

10. Reduce the amount of cleaning you undertake. Tidy and sanitary are two different ideas. Providing our kids with a clean living and learning environment is essential to their health. It's not essential to have everything put away in its correct place at all times. Children are born

to destroy, at least in the beginning, and homes are made to be occupied. So, allow yourself the odd mess and give yourself a break. Find a technique that works for you and doesn't make you feel as if you're repeating the same day. The rewards and pleasures of being a mother Being a mother suggests that you are, for the most part, always required and expected to help. It took me a while to get used to always being alert. And my worries started when I became a mother. Your kids are your first priority at all times. You worry about all the little things, about whether you are raising them well, and about if you will be able to raise them appropriately. A mother must, however, be able to let go of her mother guilt and live her life following both her own and other people's objectives. It all boils down to finding a balance and revealing to your kids that you are also a human being with flaws. that you have a distinct identity and goals in addition to being a mommy.

CHAPTER FiVE

The benefits and joys of motherhood

Being a mother implies that, for the most part, you are constantly needed and expected to provide assistance. I needed some time to adjust to always being on the lookout. And becoming a mother was the beginning of my anxieties. Your children are your constant concern. You are concerned about whether you will be able to raise them properly; you are worried about whether you are doing a good job; and you are worried about all the trivial things. However, a mother needs to be able to let go of her mother guilt and spend her life pursuing her own goals as well as those of other people. It all comes down to striking a balance and letting your children know that you are a fallible human being too. that in addition to becoming a mother, you also have a personal identity and aspirations.

Plenty of Jokes and Humour

If there are kids living there, you can know right away as you walk in the door. Children's homes are thus often lively and light-filled. Parenting never gets boring. You smile at their absurd antics and sincere efforts at showing sympathy. Occasionally, they say something that instantly puts a grin on your face and allays your anxieties. The intelligence of my children never ceases to amaze me. They open my eyes to new possibilities and make me wonder why I hadn't thought of them before. Because they can distinguish your face from everyone else's, the younger ones will smile the most. Viewing previous infant pictures of your kids might help you heal more quickly. Parenting is probably not always simple. Our identities change when we become parents. Nothing in our life will ever be the same. Do we, however, overlook the little pleasures of parenting in the middle of the challenging daily grind? Do we give them enough credit for making our lives so much more enjoyable? They give you a warm, fuzzy sensation. No matter how awful you feel about yourself, your kids love you without condition. They think that because you are everything, life would not be possible without you. Being valued gives you a sense of importance. I was pleased with myself since I was kind and understanding to other people. When I'm feeling down, I give God a quiet thank you for all the little things in my life that cheer me up and make me feel better.

YOU ALWAYS HAVE A COMPANION.

As a mother, you are never alone yourself. For parents who are introverted, it can not be easy. They are fun company, however, if you can learn to establish limits with them. You could want to notify all of your older children. And talking to your mother is the best thing ever, no matter how old you become. Do other individuals think and feel the same way I do? As they become older, mothers share everything with their kids, and kids want to share everything with their parents. You are less prone to feel bored and lonely since you have them.

Parenting is probably not always simple. Our identities change when we become parents. Nothing in our life will ever be the same. Do we, however, overlook the little pleasures of parenting in the middle of the challenging daily grind? They provide motivation for living. Having kids gives your life purpose and fulfilment. Having said that, I think a woman's aspirations should go beyond being a mother. Nevertheless, meeting your children's needs comes first in your life when you have them. It is feasible to be ready for everything at all times. When they succeed, you rejoice with them and are glad for them. Additionally, remembering your kids gets you through trying times when all you want to do is give up.Your children are what keep you going.

THEY STRENGTHEN YOUR MARRIAGE

As you begin your parenting journey together, having children helps to deepen your relationship with your partner. Born out of your mutual love, your kid is your wonderful creation.

Your kid serves as a constant link between you two, strengthening the already strong tie between you.

After having children, many individuals discover a renewed appreciation for their spouse. The spouse witnesses his spouse's transformation into a devoted father figure, while the spouse gains insight into his spouse's compassionate and resilient side.

Not everyone, but a lot of individuals like bettering themselves once they become parents. Their marriage also benefits from their being more responsible and mature adults.

Once children are involved, couples are inclined to work more at their marriage. Since it is everyone's goal to provide their children a secure and contented environment.

THEY IMPROVE YOU AS A PERSON

Being a better person is one of the advantages of being a parent. You become stronger and more altruistic. You are more organised and adopt better habits.

However, all of these alter after having children since having children takes up a certain amount of time each day. I also began getting up early to make time for other healthy habits like self-care.

And patience. I advise you to attempt having children if you believe yourself to be a patient person. Your ability to be patient will be put to the test, and you'll discover whether you really are or not.

You also develop more empathy and kindness. You have to learn to give up the negative habits if you want to be a positive role model for your children.

THEY STRENGTHEN YOUR MARRIAGE

As you begin your parenting journey together, having children helps to deepen your relationship with your partner. Born out of your mutual love, your kid is your wonderful creation. Your kid serves as a constant link between you two, strengthening the already strong tie between you. After having children, many individuals discover a renewed appreciation for their spouse. The spouse witnesses his spouse's transformation into a devoted father figure, while the spouse gains insight into his spouse's compassionate and resilient side. Not everyone, but a lot of individuals like bettering themselves once they become parents. Their marriage also benefits from their being more responsible and mature adults. Once children are involved, couples are inclined to work harder at their marriage. Since it is everyone's goal to provide their children with a secure and contented environment,

THEY IMPROVE YOU AS A PERSON

Being a better person is one of the advantages of being a parent. You become stronger and more altruistic. You are more organised and adopt better habits. However, all of these alter after having children, since having children takes up a certain amount of time each day. I also began getting up early to make time for other healthy habits, like self-care. And patience. I advise you to attempt having children if you believe yourself to be a patient person. Your ability to be patient will be put to the test, and you'll discover whether you really are or not. You also develop more empathy and kindness. You have to learn to give up the negative habits if you want to be a positive role model for your children. Because you know you'll be asked questions if you break the rules in your home, your kids hold you responsible.

YOU ACQUIRE IMPROVED TIME MANAGEMENT

It's true that raising children takes up a lot of your time, and you seldom get a break. Additionally, it improves your time management abilities. You become more adept at managing your time as you are aware that you have a limited amount of time each day to do certain chores. It's possible that parenting is not always simple. When we become mothers, we change as humans. Our lives will never be the same.

MORE THAN YOU LOVE YOUR PARENTS

You don't realise what your parents went through to raise you until you're a parent. It increases your empathy for your parents. and increases your gratitude for them. I'm not arguing that if you don't have children, you won't appreciate your parents sufficiently. Even if they are childless, I know individuals who look after their parents properly. However, you "live" the life they lived when you became a parent. And it makes it easier for you to understand the difficulties and hard work. When do you feel that you really appreciate your parents? when the negative tendencies you had as a child are still present in your children. Haha!

YOU GROW STRONG

During delivery, your body demonstrates its strength. Women are able to tolerate pain to such an extent that it increases their self-confidence in their capacity to tolerate pain. Motherhood also brings up a vast spectrum of emotions. You develop more patience, empathy, and compassion. Not to mention the disappointments, anxieties, and melancholy. You become stronger and more equipped to deal with the harsh reality of the outside world after you have experienced all the emotions. Did you ever believe as a youngster that "my mommy can fix anything"? It's not that you are an expert. However, you sort things out as you go along because you are a problem solver for your kids. You must learn to rise to every situation in order to keep your kids safe.

YOU START TO SHOW GRATEFULNESS.

Learning new things with your kids is one of the delights of being a mother. Because we have lived on this planet for such a long time, we often take minor things for granted. However, you rediscover your surroundings when you see through a child's inquisitive eyes. Children teach you the value of mindfulness and how to find joy in even the little things in life. They don't worry about the past or the future; they just live in the now. Isn't that what we learn from meditation? Perhaps children are born meditators.

A mother's and her child's relationship is a multifaceted and exquisite fabric that threads together through all of life's phases. From the precious moments of infancy to the struggles of adolescence and the deep connection in maturity, the development of the mother-child relationship is a journey distinguished by growth, resilience, and everlasting love.

I. The Precarious Origins: Infant Attachment A mother's bond with her child is like a fragile flower in its early stages. The foundation of trust and dependency is established when a baby curls up in a mother's arms. Calm lullabies respond to the baby's screams, forming a rhythmic dance of tenderness and reassurance.

II. The Dance of Exploration: Toddlerhood The mother-child bond transforms into a dance of discovery when the child enters the adventurous stage of toddlerhood. As the child takes those first steps, explores the world, and learns to love freedom, the mother acts as a guiding hand.

III. Primary Years: Promoting Development and Education During the primary school years, the mother assumes the role of an educator and advisor. The bond grows when homework assistance and encouragement for learning are provided. In addition to fostering enduring memories, shared experiences help the mother become a dependable figure in her child's self-discovery path.

IV. Adolescence: Getting Over Troubled Waters The adolescent years usher in a time of instability and change. As the kid struggles with identity and yearns for autonomy, the mother-child connection must traverse rough waters. Even if there may be conflicts, the relationship is put to the test and made stronger by honest communication, compassion, and constant support.

V. College and Independence: Letting Go When the kid grows up and maybe moves away for college, the dynamics of the relationship change significantly. The mother must struggle with the difficult task of letting go, allowing the child to choose their own path while continuing to be a distant source of support and direction.

VI. Grandparenting Completes the Circle of Motherhood The bond between a mother and her child completes a circle in later life, when the youngster may become a parent. When a mother becomes a grandmother, she passes on her knowledge, experience, and support to the next generation. The happiness of seeing one's child become a parent brings another level of development to the connection.

VII. The Difficulties of Ageing: A Shift in Roles The connection may encounter additional difficulties as the mother and child become older. As the mother matures, the once-dependent child can find themselves in a caring position. The connection takes on a new level as it develops, one that is complicated by the difficulties of shifting roles as well as the heartbreaking beauty of shared memories.

VIII. Treasured Moments: Common Customs and Recollections A treasure trove of memories, inside jokes, and shared rituals are among the precious moments that punctuate the mother-child bond throughout the voyage. Their common experiences serve as the stitches holding their relationship together, leaving a legacy that stands the test of time.

IX. The Indestructible Fibre: Lasting Love The love thread endures in spite of the relationship's changing dynamics. A mother's and child's love endures forever because it is developed through many shared moments, victories, and struggles. It's a love that changes, grows, and endures despite life's unpredictable course. The mother-child bond has grown over time via a process of adjustment, development, and unwavering love. The connection creates a tapestry that depicts a tale of shared experiences, resiliency, and love that is a monument to the wonder of the maternal link, from the frail beginnings of infancy to the complexity of maturity. When the tapestry is unrolled, a love heritage and a connection that lasts beyond time are revealed.

JUGGLING Self CARE

The numerous difficulties that come with becoming a mother may have a serious impact on mental health. Professionals provide advice on juggling parenthood with self-care. Maintaining mental health requires striking a balance between parental duties and self-care, which is particularly important for moms, who often have to juggle many tasks and responsibilities. Motherhood presents a number of difficulties that may have a substantial impact on mental health, such as lack of sleep, loneliness, and the intense pressure to live up to social expectations. Mothers need to know that looking after their mental health is not selfish but rather essential to their general wellbeing. It's crucial to learn when to say no, assign duties to others, and schedule specific time for self-care activities that encourage rest and renewal. Mothers may improve their capacity to care for their children and have healthier, more rewarding lives by making self-care a priority. Furthermore, surrounding oneself with sympathetic and understanding people, such as family, friends, or support groups, may provide chances for self-care as well as practical help, emotional support, and support. Having a support system that understands and recognises the difficulties of parenting may have a big impact. Being a mother is an amazing experience for every woman, but being pregnant may also present a lot of mental difficulties. Additionally, the mother develops sadness, mood swings, and weeping fits as a consequence of this. These women are more likely to suffer mood swings or postpartum depression after birth; it's known as anti-partum depression. Approximately 2% of expectant patients who come to our outpatient department experience depression throughout their pregnancy and need medical attention and counselling. Having supportive families at this time is crucial to these women's emotional well-being. In addition, women tend to overlook their mental health for a variety of reasons, including ignorance, laziness, an excessive workload, etc. Avoiding this is advised, as putting mental health first benefits women's general wellbeing throughout their recovery. Psychological counselling is required in cases of depressive episodes, as it will help the patient deal with emotional difficulties even more. Social pressures and expectations Aiming for Equilibrium Being a mother is a very meaningful and life-changing event that offers great happiness and contentment. But it also has its share of difficulties, and for many moms, the pressure from society is one of the biggest causes of stress. Mothers always strive to satisfy unreasonable standards while balancing many tasks as cultural norms and expectations change. A woman is inundated with idealised depictions of motherhood via the media, social media, and cultural representations as soon as she finds out she is pregnant. The image of the "perfect mother" is one of someone who effortlessly juggles her personal obligations, professional obligations, and family duties while maintaining a calm and happy demeanour. She must maintain her looks and self-care, handle her home like a pro, cook wholesome meals, participate in educational activities with her kids, and be an engaged member of the community. Unfortunately, this idealised norm is not only impractical but also impossible. Work and parenting Modern culture frequently sets a woman's work objectives against her position as a mother, causing her to make tough decisions that might lead to shame and discontent. While stay-at-home women may feel under pressure to defend their choice to put parenting above their profession, working mothers may feel guilty for not spending enough time with their kids. It may be difficult to find a balance between work and parenting, and expectations from society sometimes make things worse. The strain on moms has increased with the introduction of social media. Social media sites that were meant to foster connections have instead become hubs for mom-shaming and comparing. When mothers contrast their houses, their children's accomplishments, and their parenting methods with those shown on apparently flawless social media pages, they may feel inadequate. Anxiety and tension brought on by the dread of criticism or judgement may have a detrimental effect on one's mental health. The idea that moms should be able to manage every element of their lives with ease is perpetuated by the "Supermom" myth. Burnout and both physical and emotional tiredness may result from this strain to do everything. It's common for women to feel bad about asking for assistance or support because they think it would diminish their value as moms. In addition to harming individual moms, this irrational expectation diminishes the significance of shared tasks in childrearing and elder care. actions to make the environment more mother-supportive

Challenging Stereotypes:

We must confront the preconceived notions and expectations that are placed on moms. Reiterate that every mother's experience is different and that there is no one-size-fits-all method to parenting. Encouraging Work-Life Balance: Companies and legislators should strive to provide family-friendly work environments, provide flexible work schedules, and promote reasonably priced daycare alternatives. Encouraging shared parenting duties may empower dads by offering crucial assistance to moms and fostering a more equal home environment. Creating a Positive Community: Create a welcoming environment free from mom-shaming and judgement that embraces a variety of parenting philosophies and approaches. Making Self-Care a Priority: Help moms make self-care a priority without feeling guilty. A woman who is emotionally content and gets enough sleep is better able to be present and involved with her family.

Conclusion

The canvas of common experiences and deep insights appears before us as we approach the concluding strokes of "The Tunnel of light," serving as a monument to the timeless beauty of the maternal journey. Every chapter in this book is a vivid colour in the motherhood palette, and together they have created a work of art that lives beyond its pages. Mothers evolve as resilient creators, woven into the fabric of their lives with threads of love and commitment via the delicate skill of managing obligations and the dance of pregnancy and delivery. The emotional rollercoaster, with its euphoric highs and depressing lows, demonstrates the depth of a mother's heart as she gracefully navigates the turbulent waters. A connection that endures the test of life's many seasons is shown by examining the growth of the mother-child bond throughout time. The mother-child bond is a dynamic and timeless work of art that transcends the fragility of infancy, the complexity of adolescence, and the interplay of roles in later years. We understand that being a mother is a continuous artistic endeavour. These pages are filled with the successes of moms who have persevered in the face of hardship, encouraging us to see every obstacle as a chance for personal development. More than just a book, "The Tunnel of light" is a celebration of the power of vulnerability, the creativity that all mothers possess, and the enormous influence moms have on the course of history. With every day that goes by, every moment spent together, and every act of kindness and selflessness, the canvas is not static; it is always changing. This ending is a salute to all the mothers who have contributed to this collective work— to your unshakable commitment, your infinite love, and the everlasting imprint you leave on the canvas of life. When we take a step back and see the finished product, may it act as a timeless reminder that motherhood is a beautiful, dynamic adventure that leaves a lasting legacy of love and resilience.

www.ingramcontent.com/pod-product-compliance
Lightning Source LLC
Chambersburg PA
CBHW070750250726
48662CB00004B/1720